Dukan Diet

Easy And Delicious Consolidation And Stabilization
Phase Recipes For The Dukan Diet

(Learn How To Easily Lose Weight With The Dukan Diet)

Greg Hogan

GW00499981

TABLE OF CONTENTS

Spaghetti Squash

Ingredients

- Pepper and salt to taste
- Spaghetti squash

Direction

1. Make holes in spaghetti with knife to let out steam while cooking.
2. Now cook in the oven for about 10 minutes.
3. After cooking, allow it to cool for some time.
4. Cut lengthwise, remove seeds and then pepper and salt to taste.
5. Serve and enjoy.

Cheddar Cheese Jelly

Ingredients

- Cheddar cheese (45 0 gm)
- Jelly lite
- Boiling water

Direction

1. Blend cheese in a blender.
2. Take boiling water in a bowl and dissolve jelly in it.
3. Now add cheese to the boiling water and mix well.
4. Shift to the bowls and chill in the refrigerator until set.
5. Serve and enjoy.

Stuffed Peppers

Ingredients

- Oat bran (4 tbsp)
- 4 red peppers, cut into halves, remove seeds
- Lean beef (450 gm), minced
- 2 garlic cloves, crushed
- Paprika (2 tsp)
- 2 fresh egg

Direction

1. Preheat the oven to 450 degrees Celsius.
2. Cook the peppers in the preheated oven for about 35 minutes in a greaseproof paper lined with roasting tin until soften.
3. Prepare stuffing by combining garlic, paprika, oat bran (2 tbsp), minced

beef and fresh fresh egg together in a bowl and mix well by using fork.

4. Remove the pepper from the oven, drain water and stuff with the above mixture.

5. Splash with the remaining oat bran and bake in the oven again for about 50 minutes until the oat bran turns to brown and the meat is tender.

6. Serve and enjoy the delicious recipe.

Sage And Butternut Squash Soup

Ingredients

- 6 pints of reduced salt chicken stock
- 2 small butternut squashes, peeled, and cut into large chunks
- A handful of fresh sage leaves
- Low fat cooking spray
- 2 fresh onion, chopped
- Freshly ground black pepper

Direction

1. Preheat the oven to 300 Degrees Celsius.
2. Take a baking tray line with greaseproof paper.
3. Add butternut squash to the tray, spread sage leaves over it and then flavor it with pepper.

4. Spray the mixture with cooking spray and then cook in the preheated oven for about 50 minutes until tender.
5. Also spray a separate pan with cooking spray and cook fresh onions in it until translucent.
6. Shift the above mixture to the pan containing fresh onions and then cover.
7. Simmer for about 50 minutes and then blend in a food processor until smooth.
8. Serve with herbs and enjoy.

Baked Mussels

Ingredients:

2 -inch long ginger, peeled

4 cloves garlic, minced

2 lb mussels

2 cup less fat cream cheese

1 cup green onions, minced

Directions:

1. In a bowl, mix cream cheese and green fresh onions well. Set aside.
2. In a heavy bottomed pot placed on medium high fire, add mussels, garlic and ginger.
3. Cover and cook for 25 to 35 minutes or until most of the mussels have opened fully.
4. Turn off fire, uncover pot and let it cool for ten minutes.
5. One by one, remove the mussels and break off the empty shell and discard. Arrange shell with mussel on a baking sheet.
6. Meanwhile preheat oven to 480°F.
7. Once all mussels are on the baking sheet, place cream cheese mixture on top of mussels.
8. Ensure that you evenly place cream cheese mixture on each mussel and

cover it with the cream cheese mixture well.

9. Pop mussels in the oven and bake for 45 to 50 minutes or until cream cheese are melted and bubbly.

10.   Remove from oven; let it rest for 25 minutes before serving.

Oat Bran Muffin

Ingredients:

2 fresh egg s

4 tsps reduced fat, no sugar added cocoa powder

6 tbsps oat bran

2 tbsp Truvia

2 tsp baking powder

6 tbsps zero fat yogurt

Directions:

1. Preheat oven to 480ºF and line a muffin pan with muffin wrapper.
2. In a medium bowl, mix all dry ingredients together, except for Truvia.

3. In a small bowl, whisk fresh fresh egg s and yogurt until well incorporated.
4. Add truvia to the fresh fresh egg s and mix until dissolved.
5. Pour fresh fresh egg mixture into bowl of dry ingredients and whisk well to incorporate.
6. Evenly pour batter into 6 muffin lines. Pop into the oven and bake for 45 to 50 minutes or until cooked when toothpick is inserted in the middle no batter sticks to it.
7. Remove from oven, let it cool before serving.

Meringue

Ingredients:

2 tsp cream of tartar

4 fresh fresh egg whites

2 cup of Truvia

Directions:

1. Prepare fresh fresh egg whites and place at room temperature for an hour.
2. In a big bowl, whisked fresh fresh egg whites and cream of tartar until soft peaks form.
3. Slowly add sugar, one tablespoon at a time, while continuously whisking fresh fresh egg whites.

4. Preheat oven to 430oF and grease a baking sheet with cooking spray.
5. Transfer fresh fresh egg whites into a piping bag and pipe icing onto prepared pan 2 -inch apart.
6. Pop in the oven and bake until meringues are crisp and dry around 50 minutes.
7. Remove from oven, let it cool for 50 minutes before serving.

Oat Bran Cookies

Ingredients:

1/7 tsp salt

1 tsp baking soda

¾ cup oat bran

2 tbsps skim milk

2 packets Splenda

2 tbsps Splenda brown sugar

Directions:

1. Preheat oven to 490ºF and grease baking sheet.
2. Blend Splenda, brown sugar, baking soda and oat bran in a food processor.
3. Pour into bowl and mix in milk. Whisk thoroughly.

4. Spray cooking spray on batter for a second. Mix well.
5. Spoon batter into baking sheet into 2 or 2 inch circles. Pop in the oven and bake for 10 minutes.
6. Remove from oven, let it cool and enjoy.

Ginger And Oat Bran Biscuits

Ingredients:

6 tbsps zero fat quark

4 tbsps oat bran

4 beaten fresh fresh egg whites

2 tbsp Truvia

6 tsps dried ginger

Directions:

1. In a medium bowl, mix well truvia, quark, oat bran, fresh fresh egg whites and ginger.
2. The consistency of the batter should be thicker than a pancake.
3. On medium fire, place a nonstick skillet and grease with cooking spray.

4. Drop batter by spoonful around the skillet to create biscuit sized shapes.
5. Cook for 5-10 minutes per side or until desired brownness is reached.
6. You would need to cook all biscuits in batches and let it cool before storing in an air tight container.

Cappuccino Flavored Dukan Frappe

Ingredients:

35 ice cubes

4 tsps Truvia

2 cup cold skimmed milk

2 cup strong black coffee, cold

Directions:

1. In a blender, except for the ice cubes blend all ingredients together until foamy.
2. Add ice cubes and continue to blend until ice is crushed into small pieces.
3. Transfer to two serving glasses, serve and enjoy.

Fro-Yo

Ingredients:

4 tsps strawberry flavored sugar free jelly

2 large tub of fat-free natural yogurt (6 00g)

4 tbsps boiling water

Directions:

1. In a small bowl mix jelly and boiling water.
2. Mix until jelly is totally dissolved.
3. Set aside to cool for two minutes.
4. Then in a blender, blend jelly syrup and yogurt until smooth and creamy.
5. Blend well so that jelly and yogurt are incorporated well in order to avoid jelly lumps once your yogurt ice cream freezes.
6. Once you are done blending the mixture thoroughly, place in a lidded container and freeze for 4 hours before serving.

Grilled Lamb Chops

Ingredients:

2 tsp black pepper

2 tsps salt

1 cup distilled white vinegar

2 lbs lamb chops

2 fresh onion, sliced thinly

2 tbsp garlic minced

Directions:

1. In a re-sealable bag, mix fresh onion, garlic, pepper, salt and vinegar. Seal the bag and shake until salt is dissolved.
2. Add lamb chops into the bag and marinate in the ref for at least two hours. While ensuring that you turn

bag after an hour to ensure that all sides are marinated well.

3. On medium high fire, preheat grill and grease grate with cooking spray.

4. Remove lamb chops from bag and cover bony ends with foil.

5. Place on the grate and grill for at least 4 minutes per side or until desired doneness is reached.

6. Remove from grill, transfer to plate, serve and enjoy.

Beef Kebabs

Ingredients:

2 tbsps Dijon mustard

1 cup low sodium soy sauce

2 tbsp cider vinegar

2 4oz Beef fillet

1 tsp thyme

2 bay leaf

1 cup fresh lemon juice

Directions:

1. Cut beef into 2 -inch cubes.
2. In a bowl, mix remaining ingredients thoroughly.
3. Add meat to seasoning mixture and marinade for at least two hours inside the ref. Ensure that you flip

meat after an hour to marinate all sides of the meat.

4. Skewer the beef in Barbecue sticks and discard marinade.

5. Place kebabs in preheated grill on medium high fire and grill for 4 to 25 minutes per sie or until desired doneness.

6. Remove from grill, let it rest for 25 minutes before serving.

Chicken Curry

Ingredients:

2 tsp paprika

2 tsp ground cinnamon

4 tbsps curry powder

2 cloves garlic, minced

2 small fresh onion, chopped

4 tbsps olive oil

2 cup water

2 tsp cayenne pepper

2 lemon, juiced

2 cup zero fat yogurt

2 tomato, sliced into wedges

2 skinless, boneless chicken breast halves, cut into ½-inch cubes

salt to taste

2 tsp truvia

2 tsp grated fresh ginger

2 bay leaf

Directions:

1. In a large nonstick sauce pan greased with cooking spray on medium high fire add fresh onion and tomatoes.
2. Stir fry for 4 minutes or until lightly wilted. Add salt, truvia, ginger, bay leaf, paprika, cinnamon, curry powder and garlic. Stir fry for 2 minutes.
3. Add chicken breasts and stir fry for 25 minutes .
4. Add 2 cup of water, cover and cook for another 50 to 35 minutes.
5. Add yogurt, cook until heated through.
6. Remove from pan, serve and enjoy.

Meat Loaf

Ingredients:

2 fresh egg s

2 tbsp Worcestershire sauce

6 pounds ground beef

2 tbsp garlic pepper seasoning

2 tbsp garlic salt

6 tbsps chili powder

Directions:

1. Preheat oven to 490ºF and grease a loaf pan with cooking spray.

27

2. Mix fresh egg s, Worcestershire sauce and ground beef in a large bowl.
3. Season with garlic pepper, garlic salt, and chili powder. Mix well again.
4. Place mixture into greased loaf pan and press to form a loaf.
5. Pop in the oven and bake for 450 minutes .
6. Remove from oven and let it stand for minutes before serving and slicing.

Tofu Stir Fry

Ingredients:

2 lime

2 tsps minced fresh ginger root

2 tsps minced garlic

2 lbs firm tofu

2 tbsp tamari

Directions:

1. On medium high fire, place a medium nonstick sauce pan and grease with cooking spray.
2. Stir fry ginger and garlic for two minutes.
3. Add tamari and tofu. Stir to mix.
4. Cover pan and lower fire to medium and cook for 35 to 50 minutes while ensuring to stir every 25 minutes .
5. Remove from pan and transfer to serving bowl.
6. Squeeze lime juice on top and serve.

Roasted Rack Of Lamb

Ingredients:

1 tsp black pepper

2 tsp salt

2 tbsps chopped fresh rosemary

2 tbsps minced garlic

2 tbsp Dijon mustard

2 tsp black pepper

2 tsp salt

2 8 -bone rack of lamb, trimmed and frenched

Directions:

1. Preheat oven to 46 0ºF.
2. In a medium bowl, mix pepper, salt, rosemary and garlic. Add 2   tbsp

water to wet ingredients and smear all around lamb rack.

3. On an oven proof nonstick skillet place on high fire, sear lamb for two minutes per side. Turn off fire.

4. Cover bony edges of lamb with foil and pop into the oven.

5. Cook for 35 to 35 minutes or until desired doneness.

6. Remove from oven and let it stand for 50 minutes before serving.

Tandoori Chicken Fillets

Ingredients:

2 tbsps zero fat yogurt

2 tbsps Tandoori Masala Spice mix

2 skinless chicken breast fillets

2 -cm piece of peeled ginger

2 garlic clove

2 green chilli

2 lemon, juiced

Directions:

1. In a food processor, blend ginger, garlic, green chili, lemon juice, yogurt and masala spice mix until smooth.
2. Score chicken two or three times per piece to allow flavors to seep in.

3. Place seasoning mixture into a bowl and add chicken. Toss well to mix. Cover with cling wrap and let it sit in the ref for a night.
4. Grill chicken for 10 to 15 minutes per side or until desired doneness is achieved.
5. Serve with a side of zero fat yogurt.

Mexican Chicken

INGREDIENTS

6 tsp cumin

2 tsp cayenne pepper

2 tsp paprika

2 tsp oil

2 chicken breasts

2 bell peppers

2 cups broccoli florets

DIRECTIONS

1. Heat a pan

2. Heat the oil for about 35 seconds

3. Add diced chicken and cook for 25 minutes

4. Add the broccoli and peppers and cook for another 35 minutes

5. Add the spices
6. Cook until the water is absorbed

Grilled Salmon

INGREDIENTS

- 6 tbs oil
- 2 tsp fresh onion powder
- 2 tsp chili powder
- 2 avocado
- 2 tsp salt
- 2 red fresh onion
- 2 limes juiced
- 2 tbs cilantro
- 6 tsp cumin
- 6 tsp paprika
- 2 lbs salmon

DIRECTIONS

1. Mix the chili powder, fresh onion powder, cumin, paprika, salt and pepper together
2. Rub the salmon with the mix and oil
3. Refrigerate for 50 minutes
4. Preheat the grill
5. Mix the avocado with lime juice, cilantro, and fresh onion together
6. Grill the salmon
7. Serve topped with the avocado salsa

Cuban Quinoa

INGREDIENTS

- 2 cup corn
- 2 cup quinoa
- 2 tsp garlic
- 2 can tomatoes
- 2 jalapeno
- 2 cups enchilada sauce
- 6 cup chicken broth
- 2 can black beans
- 2 lb butternut squash

DIRECTIONS

1. Peel and deseed the butternut squash
2. Cut into cubes, then place in the slow cooker

3. Add the corn, quinoa, garlic, tomatoes, black beans, jalapeno, enchilada sauce and the chicken broth

4. Give it a good stir, then cook for 4 hours

5. Allow the liquid to absorb while on low for 50 minutes

6. Season with salt and pepper

Roasted Squash

INGREDIENTS

- 2 tsp curry powder
- 2 tsp salt
- 2 delicata squashes
- 2 tablespoons olive oil

DIRECTIONS

1. Preheat the oven to 46 0F

2. Cut everything in half lengthwise

3. Toss everything with olive oil and place onto a prepared baking sheet

4. Roast for 40-45 minutes at 46 0F or until golden brown

5. When ready remove from the oven and serve

41

Brussels Sprout Chips

INGREDIENTS

- 2 lb. brussels sprouts
- 2 tsp garlic powder
- 2 tsp seasoning
- 2 tablespoon olive oil
- 2 tablespoon parmesan cheese

DIRECTIONS

1. Preheat the oven to 46 0F

2. In a bowl toss everything with olive oil and seasoning

3. Spread everything onto a prepared baking sheet

4. Bake for 30-35 minutes or until crisp

5. When ready remove from the oven and serve

Zucchini Chips

INGREDIENTS

- 2 tsp garlic powder
- 2 tsp seasoning
- 2 lb. zucchini
- 2 tablespoon olive oil
- 2 tablespoon parmesan cheese

DIRECTIONS

1. Preheat the oven to 46 0F

2. In a bowl toss everything with olive oil and seasoning

3. Spread everything onto a prepared baking sheet

4. Bake for 30-35 minutes or until crisp
5. When ready remove from the oven and serve

Carrot Chips

INGREDIENTS

- 2 tsp garlic powder
- 2 tsp seasoning
- 2 lb. carrot
- 2 tablespoon olive oil
- 2 tablespoon parmesan cheese

DIRECTIONS

1. Preheat the oven to 46 0F

2. In a bowl toss everything with olive oil and seasoning

3. Spread everything onto a prepared baking sheet
4. Bake for 30-35 minutes or until crisp
5. When ready remove from the oven and serve

Simple Spaghetti

INGREDIENTS

- 2 tsp black pepper
- Olive oil
- 2 tsp parsley
- 2 cloves garlic
- 35 oz. spaghetti
- 2 fresh fresh egg s
- 2 cup parmesan cheese

DIRECTIONS

1. In a pot boil spaghetti   drain and set aside

2. In a bowl whish fresh fresh egg s with parmesan cheese

3. In a skillet heat olive oil, add garlic and cook for 20-25 minutes

4. Pour fresh fresh egg mixture and mix well

5. Add pasta and stir well

6. When ready garnish with parsley and serve

Corn Pasta

INGREDIENTS

- 2 cloves garlic
- 2 tsp cumin
- 2 cups corn kernels
- 2 tsp chili powder
- 2 tablespoon cilantro
- 2 lb. pasta
- 4 oz. cheese
- 1 sour cream
- 2 fresh onion

DIRECTIONS

1. In a pot boil spaghetti, drain and set aside
2. Place all the ingredients for the sauce in a pot and bring to a simmer
3. Add pasta and mix well
4. When ready garnish with parmesan cheese and serve

Artichoke Pasta

INGREDIENTS

- 2 lb. pasta
- 2 tablespoons butter
- 2 . Cup basil
- 2 cup parmesan cheese
- 1 cup olive oil
- 2 jar artichokes
- 2 cloves garlic
- 2 tablespoon thyme leaves

DIRECTIONS

1. In a pot boil spaghetti (or any other type of pasta), drain and set aside

2. Place all the ingredients for the sauce in a pot and bring to a simmer

3. Add pasta and mix well

49

4. When ready garnish with parmesan cheese and serve

Slaw

INGREDIENTS

- 2 cabbage
- 2 bunch of baby carrots
- 2 cucumber
- 2 bun of cilantro
- 2 bunch of basil
- 2 fresh onion

DIRECTIONS

1. In a bowl combine all ingredients together and mix well
2. Serve with dressing

Sriracha Dressing

INGREDIENTS

- 2 fresh fresh egg
- 1 cup rice vinegar
- 2 tablespoon coconut aminos
- 2 tablespoon sriracha
- 2 tablespoon maple syrup

DIRECTIONS

1. In a bowl combine all ingredients together and mix well
2. Serve with dressing

Sage And Butternut Squash Soup

Ingredients:

- Cooking spray, low-fat
- Fresh onion, sliced, 2
- Oat bran galettes, her-flavored, 2 (optional)
- Black pepper
- Chicken stock, low-sodium, 6 pints
- Butternut squashes, peeled and chunked in large, 2 small
- Sage leaves, handful

Instructions:

1. Prepare oven at 300 C.
2. Add butternut squash to baking sheet line with greaseproof sheet; scatter

sage leave onto it and season with pepper.

3. Brush with cooking spray and bake in oven for about 50 minutes.

4. Fry fresh onions in a separate pan coated with cooking spray until translucent.

5. Arrange mixture alongside onions; cover with lid and simmer for about 50 minutes.

6. Arrange the food in a food processor to process until smooth before you serve alongside herbs.

Stuffed Peppers

Ingredients:

- Garlic cloves, crushed, 2
- Paprika, 2 tsp
- Fresh egg , 2
- Oat bran, 4 tbsp
- Red peppers, halved and seeds removed, 4
- Lean beef, minced, 450 gm

Instructions:

1. Prepare oven at 450 C.
2. Arrange peppers onto baking tray lined with greaseproof sheet; bake for about 35 minutes or until soften.
3. Take a bowl; add fresh egg , minced beef, 2 tbsp oat bran, paprika as well as garlic and mix using fork.

4. Separate pepper; drain and stuff alongside mixture.
5. Sprinkle with remaining oat bran and prepare for about half an hour or until meat is golden before you serve.

Cheddar Cheese Jelly

Ingredients:

Jelly lite

Boiling water

Cheddar cheese, 45 0 gm

Instructions:

Add cheese to a food processor and process well.

Dissolve jelly in boiling water.

Put cheese in boiling water as well and combine.

Arrange in a bowl and let it stand in refrigerator before you serve.

Spaghetti Squash

Ingredients:

Salt and pepper to taste
Spaghetti squash

Instructions:

1. Let the steam out through piercing in spaghetti meanwhile it cooks.
2. Cook for about 25 minutes .
3. Let it stand for a while afterwards.
4. Vertically chop; separate the seeds and sprinkle with salt as well as pepper before you serve.

Oat Bran Granola

Ingredients:

Oat bran, 2 tbsp

Syrup, sugar free

Instructions:

1. Add syrup as well as oat bran in a bowl and combine.
2. Microwave it for about 2 minutes and separate afterwards.
3. Keep it aside to cool before you serve with yogurt.

Petits Pains D'avoine

Ingredients:

- Cream cheese, fat-free, 2 tbsp
- Baking powder, 2 tsp
- Yogurt, fat-free, 2 cup
- Oat bran
- Fresh egg s, 2

Instructions:

1. Prepare oven at 300 C.
2. Take a bowl; add all ingredients to it and combine until smooth.
3. Place mixture onto baking sheet and bake for about 35 minutes before you serve.

Salmon With Ginger

Ingredients:

Ginger to taste

Garlic cloves, 2

Soy sauce, low-sodium

Salmon fillet, 2

Instructions:

1. Prepare oven at 45 0 C.
2. Add salmon with all other ingredients in a dish; cover with foil and pierce.
3. Bake in oven for about 50 minutes before you serve.

Beef Stew

Ingredients:

- Celery sticks, roughly sliced, 4
- Black pepper to taste
- Carrots, chopped medium, 2
- Lean beef, strips, 480 gm
- Corn flour, 2 tbsp
- Oregano, dried, 2 tsp
- Cooking spray, low-fat
- Bay leaves, 2
- Dried thyme, 2 tsp
- Chesnut mushrooms, chopped, 8
- Beef stock, low-sodium, 6 pint
- Shallots, peeled, 450 gm

Instructions:

1. Prepare oven at 450 C.
2. Add corn flour alongside beef with splashed pepper to coat.
3. Add carrots, shallots, celery, herbs as well as mushrooms in a bowl; combine and keep it aside.
4. Cook beef in a pan coated with cooking spray and cook until golden.
5. Arrange beef onto a casserole dish alongside vfresh egg ies and wrap.
6. Bake for about 2 hours or until stock thickens before you serve.

Chicken Shirataki Noodle Soup

Ingredients:

Corn flour, 2 tbsp, melted in 2 tbsp of water

Celery sticks, sliced, 4

Spring onions, sliced, 4

Cooking spray, low-fat

Carrot, sliced, 2 medium

Shirataki noodles, 35 0 gm

Soy sauce, low-sodium, 2 tbsp

Chicken, cooked, 300 gm

Mange tout, 450 gm

Courgette, chopped, 2 medium

All spice, 2 tsp

Chicken stock, low-sodium, 6 pints

Ginger, grated, 2 tsp

Instructions:

1. Prepare noodles in hot water and transfer it to cooking dish alongside hot boiled water.
2. Let it stand for about 2 minutes; rinse and keep it aside afterwards.
3. Add celery, carrot as well as spring fresh onion in a saucepan coated with cooking spray and cook for about 4 minutes or until translucent.
4. Add ginger and simmer for about half a minute.
5. Now add spice, mange tout, corn flour, courgette as well as chicken stock and simmer for 45-50 more minutes.
6. Add soy sauce alongside shirataki noodles and simmer for about 4 more minutes before you serve.

Curried Cauliflower Soup

Ingredients:

Coriander, 2 tsp

Ginger, grated, 2 tsp

Curry powder, 2 tsp

Fresh onion, thinly sliced, 2 small

Garlic, thinly sliced, 2 cloves

Cauliflower, roughly sliced, 2 small head

Cooking spray, low-fat

Oat bran galettes, herb-flavored, 2

Chili powder, 2 tsp

Vegetable stock, low-salt, 6 pints

Cumin, 2 tsp

Instructions:

1. Take a bowl; add garlic, 2 tbsp water, spices as well as ginger and combine.
2. Fry fresh onion in a saucepan coated with cooking spray until translucent.
3. Add curry paste and simmer for about 2 more minute.
4. Add cauliflower followed by vegetable stock; cover with cauliflower and simmer for about 50 minutes.
5. Separate it from the pan; process mixture and enjoy with favorite hers as well as oat bran.

Kale And Blueberry Smoothie

Ingredients:

Ice cubes, 6

Blueberries, frozen, 2 cup

Almond butter, 2 tbsp

Yogurt, non-fat, 2 up

Kales, handful

Instructions:

1. In a food processor; add all ingredients together and blend until smooth before you serve.

Red Pepper Fajitas And Chili Chicken

Ingredients:

Oat bran, 4 tbsp

Greek yogurt, 4 tbsp

Fresh egg s, 2

Oat Bran Galette:
Chili pepper, thinly sliced and seeds removed, 2

Dried thyme, 2 tsp

Chili Chicken:

Chicken breasts, 2 small

Red peppers, 2

Parsley, sliced, handful

Cream cheese, low-fat

Fresh onion, 2 small

Hot chili powder, 2 tsp

Instructions:

2. Combine thyme, green chili alongside oat bran; cook and keep it aside.
3. prepare griddle pan on medium high heat for about 10 minutes.
4. Take a bowl; add sliced chicken, pepper as well as fresh onion and combine.
5. Add chili powder and spoon well.

6. Arrange chicken as well as vfresh egg ies onto pan and cook until tender.
7. Distribute oat bran onto platter and scatter cream cheese onto it.
8. Arrange chicken onto it and serve with parsley topping.

Tomato Fresh Egg S

Ingredients:

Fresh onion, sliced, 2

Cooking spray

Fresh egg s, 4

Salt and pepper

Basil leaves, roughly sliced, few

Tomatoes, sliced, 46 0gm

Warm water, 4 tbsp

Instructions:

1. Fry fresh onion in a saucepan coated with cooking spray for few minutes or until translucent on medium high heat.
2. Add 4 tbsp of water as well as tomatoes; mix and cook for about 50 minutes.
3. Add mixture with basil and combine until absorbed.
4. Add broken fresh fresh egg s onto mixture and serve with sprinkled pepper as well as salt.

Chicken Greek Salad

Ingredients:

Lettuce, 2 little

Red pepper, diced, 2

Chicken, cooked, 450 gm

Cucumber, diced, peeled, 2

Red fresh onion, thinly sliced, 2 small

Cooking spray

Dried oregano, 2 tbsp

Tomatoes, diced, 4 medium

Instructions:

1. Add all ingredients to a shallow bowl alongside cooking spray and combine before you serve.

Chicken Mince Mushrooms

Ingredients:

Natural yogurt, low-fat, 4 tbsp

Boiling water, 2 45 ml

Chestnuts mushrooms, quartered, 8

Red fresh onion, sliced, 2

Chicken, minced, 600 gm

Canned tomatoes, sliced, 800 gm

Salt, 2 tsp

Olive oil, 2 tbsp

Chili con carne spice mix, 2 packet

Instructions:

2. Prepare oven at 450 C.
3. Take a bowl; add all ingredients and whisk to mix.
4. Transfer it to a casserole dish.
5. Cover with lid and bake in oven for about 2 hour and 50 minutes; spoon often.
6. Add yogurt before you serve.

Sea Bass Fillets With Oat Bran Crust

Ingredients:

Olive oil

Parsley, thinly sliced, handful

Sea bass fillets, 4

Oat bran, 4 tbsp

Few sprigs of thyme

Black pepper

Water, 2 tbsp

Instructions:

1. Prepare oven at 450 C.
2. Take a bowl; add oat bran, herb, bread crumbs as well as water and mix.

3. Brush breadcrumb mixture onto each fillet and arrange on to baking sheet coated with cooking spray.
4. Bake in oven for about 30 minutes before you serve.

Chilli And Ginger Roast Chicken

Ingredients
<u>Ingredients</u>

2 teaspoon of paprika

4 cloves of garlic

2 teaspoons of dried oregano

2 fresh lemon

2 whole medium-sized chicken

2 cube of fresh ginger red chilli pepper

Instructions

1. Pre-heat the oven to 30 0 0 degrees C or 300 if your oven does not have a fan.
2. Cut fresh lemon into two halves, dent the fresh lemon , squeeze some of the juice into the cavity of the chicken,

and press the fresh lemon halves inside.

3. Find a roasting tin to put the chicken.

4. Remove the green stalk and ends of the red chilli, slice it at the middle and remove the seeds.

5. Cut into small pieces and put into the roasting tin with the chicken breast.

6. Peel and cut the ginger into small equal pieces.

7. Divide each of the 4 garlic cloves along their length.

8. Stab the chicken breast with a sharp knife to make room for the ginger, garlic and chilli.

9. Sprinkle the oregano and paprika on the top.

10. Place in the oven for 4 hours to cook until the chicken is set and turns brown.

11. Once cooked, remove the chicken and cut it; ensure that that there is no

blood and the juices are clear and
then serve.

Fresh Lemon Chicken Skewers

Ingredients

For the marinade:

2 cube of fresh sliced ginger

2 Large sliced clove of garlic A handful
of fresh chopped coriander

2 chopped red chilli Juice of one fresh
lemon

For the dip:

- 2 teaspoon of paprika
- 2 tablespoons of chopped fresh
  chives

- 2 tablespoons of chopped fresh parsley
- 45 og of fat free Greek yogurt

- Salt and pepper

Instructions

3. Mix all the marinade ingredients in a bowl.
4. Chop the chicken breasts into chunks. Add them to the marinade, stir to mix well, and then cover with cling film. Put in the fridge to marinate for at least half an hour. You can leave it for an hour or more for best results if you have the time.

5. Prepare the dip by mixing all the ingredients in a small bowl, add a pinch of salt and pepper to taste, and then refrigerate while the chicken is marinating.
6. Cook in the oven under medium grill for about twenty-five minutes until it turns golden brown.
7. Serve with the parsley dip and dill.

Caraway Flavored Pork Chops

Ingredients

- 2 fresh lemon
- Salt and pepper to taste
- 2 pork chops
- 2 tablespoon of caraway seeds

Instructions

4. Heat the oven to 2 8o degrees C. Remove any visible fats from the pork chops using a chopping board and put on a plate.
5. Crush the caraway seeds into powder using a pestle and mortar then sprinkle around the pork chops then add salt and pepper to taste.

6. Sauté the meat using a slightly greased non-stick pan under medium heat.

7. Put the pork chops in a roasting tin once they are set and have turned brown.

8. Let it cook and squeeze the fresh lemon juice around the pork chops and serve.

Thai Chicken Patties

Ingredients

For the chicken patties:

- 4 tablespoons of fresh coriander
- 2 green, roughly chopped chilli
- 2 red onion chopped
- 2 chopped garlic clove
- 2 small, peeled and chopped piece of fresh ginger
- 480g of ground chicken
- For the dip:
- 2 tablespoons of chopped fresh chives
- 45 og of 0% fat Greek yogurt
- A splash of fresh lemon juice
- 4 chopped spring onions
- Salt and black pepper to taste

Instructions

4. Prepare the dip by mixing all the ingredients in a food processor or blender, add salt and pepper to taste and puree until smooth. Pour into a small bowl, and use a cling film to cover. Put in the fridge while you prepare the chicken patties.

5. Put all the Thai patties ingredients except the chicken in a food processor and blend. Pour these ingredients into the chicken and mix thoroughly. Mould six small cakes using your hand.

6. Cook the patties in a lightly greased non-stick pan under medium heat until they turn golden brown. This can take ten minutes.

7. Serve with the Greek yogurt dip.

Steak Pizzaiola

Ingredients

- Cooking spray to grease the pan
- A handful of chopped flat leaf parsley
- Black pepper to taste
- 2 lean beef frying steaks or veal escalopes
- 2 sliced cloves of garlic
- 2 tablespoons of tomato paste

Instructions

6. Dilute the tomato paste with a few tablespoons of warm water in a small bowl then grease the frying pan with the cooking spray and put the veal escalopes, without the hob, in the pan.

7. Daub the tomato paste around the meat, and then add garlic to top, with half of the chopped parsley. Let this cook for around fifteen minutes over medium heat or until they are properly cooked.

8. Add some hot water if the tomato sauce gets too thick while cooking. Add freshly ground black pepper when the steaks are done, and then sprinkle with the rest of the chopped parsley and serve when hot.

Spanish Sea Food

Ingredients

- A few drops of extra-virgin olive oil
- 2 packet of refrigerated and pre-cooked seafood mix (prawns, mussels, squid)
- 2 teaspoon of tomato puree
- 2 clove of finely chopped or crushed garlic Chopped chives
- 2 chopped red chilli Salt and pepper to taste

Instructions

7. Put the extra virgin oil in a pan then let it melt under medium heat and add the garlic.

8. Add the seafood when the garlic has browned. Bring them to a boil then add chili, salt, and pepper to taste.

9. Let these cook for 10 minutes before you add the tomato puree.
10. Leave for another 10 minutes to cook then top with the chives and serve.

Tuna And Tzatzild Sauce

Ingredients

- 2 tuna steaks
- For the marinade
- Juice of one lime
- 2 tablespoons of teriyaki sauce
- Black pepper to taste
- For the tzatziki
- 1/2 of a de-seeded and roughly chopped cucumber
- 45 og o% fat Greek yogurt
- Juice of one lime
- 2 clove of crushed garlic
- Salt and pepper to taste
- 2 tablespoons of chopped fresh dill

Instructions

8. Mix the teriyaki sauce in a small bowl with the limejuice.
9. Dip the tuna steaks in the bowl, and roll them until they are fully covered in the marinade.
10. Put in the fridge to cool for at least 45 minutes but make sure to cover with cling film.
11. Prepare the dip before the thirty minutes are up by blending the garlic, cucumber, fresh lemon juice and dill in a blender or food processor until a smooth mixture is formed.

12. Pour Greek yogurt into a bowl, and then blend in with the cucumber paste. Cover with cling film and refrigerate.

13. Once you have marinated the chicken enough, remove from the

fridge then spray a non stick pan with oil spray and place over medium heat and then add the tuna steaks. Depending on your cooking preferences, you can sear for around two minutes if you want it fairly red, or more if you want it thoroughly cooked.

14. Be sure not to overcook it though. Remove the tzatziki dip and serve with the tuna.

Mini Burgers

Ingredients

- 2 tablespoons of oat bran
- 2 small chopped cloves of garlic
- 2 green chilli, chopped (optional)
- 2 fresh egg
- 600g of lean turkey mince
- 2 tablespoon of Cajun spice mix

Instructions

9. Blend in the mince with the rest of the ingredients in a bowl using a fork. You can use a food processor if you have it to speed up things.
10. Shape the turkey mixture using your hands to get eight small burgers. Place a griddle pan over medium heat and preheat it for about five minutes.

11. Arrange the burgers on the griddle pan, and let them cook until they are done and the meat is cooked.

12. Best served hot with 0% fat Greek yogurt.

Rosemary Beef Burgers

Ingredients

For the burgers

- 4 tablespoons of oat bran
- Freshly ground black pepper
- 2 teaspoon of nutmeg
- 2 whole fresh egg
- 46 og lean beef mince
- 2 tablespoons of chopped fresh rosemary
- For the dip:
- 45 og of 0% fat Greek yogurt
- 2 teaspoons of dried dill
- 2 teaspoon of smoked paprika

Instructions

1. Blend in all the ingredients for the yogurt dip in a bowl then cover with cling film and set in the fridge to cool.

2. Mix the rest of the ingredients for the burgers in a food processor, or in a bowl with a fork if you do not have the processor.

3. Make ten burgers from the mixture by molding using your hands.   Place a griddle pan over high heat and let it heat up for about five minutes. Place your burgers on the griddle pan then let them cook until the burgers turn brown and the meat is well cooked.

4. Serve hot with the dill and paprika dip.

Salmon Baked Omelet

Ingredients

- 2oog smoked salmon
- 6 fresh egg s
- 2 tablespoons of fat-free natural yogurt
- 2 tablespoon of chopped fresh chives
- 2 tablespoon of dried dill
- Freshly ground black pepper

Instructions

1. Pre-heat the oven to 450 degrees C.
2. Chop the smoked salmon roughly then set 2/4 aside to use with the fresh egg s, and the remaining 1/2 to top the omelet.
3. Mix the yogurt, dried drill and the fresh egg s in a bowl.

4. Add the chopped salmon, and mix well. Add the freshly ground black pepper to season.

5. Pour the fresh egg mixture into a tin mold made of silicone so that you don't use any extra fat and the omelet does not stick to the mold.

6. Place the remaining salmon close together at the top of the omelet, and add the chopped chives at the top.

7. Place in the oven for about forty minutes to cook.

8. Serve.

Turkey Kebabs

Ingredients

- Juice of 2 fresh lemon
- 2 teaspoon of turmeric
- 2 teaspoon of ground ginger
- 1/2 teaspoon of saffron
- 2 teaspoon of black pepper
- 6 oog of diced turkey thigh (or chicken breast)
- 2 teaspoons of paprika
- 2 cloves of crushed garlic

Instructions

1. Strip the turkey cubes of any visible fat and put them in a bowl. Add the rest of the ingredients, and blend them in using your hands to make sure that each piece of meat is

covered with the spice mixture. Put this in the fridge for about one hour to marinate but be sure to cover the bowl with a cling film. The longer it stays chilled, the better the results.

2. Put the kebabs together using metal or bamboo skewers and place them aside.

3. Place a griddle pan under high heat for about five minutes before you put the kebabs. Let them cook until the meat is done and turns golden brown.

Salmon And Cream Cheese Wrap

Ingredients

- 2 tablespoon of low fat cream cheese
- 4 tablespoons of oat bran
- 2 chives flavored oat bran galette
- 2 whole fresh egg s or fresh egg whites
- A few slices of smoked salmon
- 4 tablespoons of 0% fat Greek yogurt
- Black pepper

Instructions

1. Mix all the ingredients in a bowl using a whisk until a smooth batter forms. Add a little yogurt if the batter comes

out too thick. Add one tablespoon of chopped chives to the mixture.

2. Lightly grease the bottom of a non-stick pan and pour half of the batter. Place the pan over medium heat until the pancake turns golden brown on all sides. Remove and repeat this process for the second pancake.

3. Let the pancake stay for a couple of minutes to cool down. Press the cream cheese on the galette and top with the smoked salmon. Add black pepper to season.

4. Fold and seal the wraps then slice halfway and enjoy.

Bacon And Scrambled Fresh Egg S Sandwich

Ingredients

2 oat bran galettes 4 fresh egg s
2 pack of turkey bacon rashers
A pinch of dried dill
4 tablespoons of skimmed milk Salt and pepper
For the pancakes
2 whole fresh egg s or fresh egg whites
4 tablespoons of 0% fat Greek yogurt 4 tablespoons of oat bran

Instructions for the pancakes

1. Mix all the ingredients in a bowl using a whisk until a smooth batter forms.

105

Add a little yogurt if the batter comes out too thick.

2. Lightly grease the bottom of a non-stick pan and pour half of the batter in. Place the pan over medium heat until the pancake turns golden brown on all sides. Remove and repeat this process for the second pancake, place on a plate and cover to keep warm.

3. Instructions for the scrambled fresh egg s mix

4. Break 4 fresh egg s into a bowl, and add the skimmed milk. Whisk the mixture together until the milk and fresh egg s have blended. Add salt and pepper to taste, and then sprinkle with a pinch of dried dill. If you do not use dill, you can use any herb of your choice such as tarragon as a replacement.

5. Spray a non-stick pan with vegetable oil spray and place it under medium

heat for a few minutes. Add the fresh egg mixture when the pan is hot enough, allow it to cook for a couple of minutes, and then pull the fresh egg s on the edges to the center with a spatula. Fold the fresh egg s until they are done but moist.

6. Spray another non slick pan with vegetable oil spray then place it under medium heat and fry the turkey rashers.

7. Place them on the pancakes then add the scrambled fresh egg s at the top, and then make two sandwiches by folding the oat bran galettes.

8. Serve hot.

Oat Bran Galette With Toffee Yogurt Ingredients

- 2 tablespoons of oat bran
- 2 fresh egg
- 2 teaspoon of sweetener
- 2 tablespoons of 0% fat Greek yogurt
- 2 small pot of low fat toffee yogurt

Instructions

1. Start by first mixing the oat bran, fresh egg , sweetener and yogurt until smooth.
2. Lightly grease a non-stick pan and place it under medium heat until hot. Pour in half of the mixture and cook the pancake on both sides until golden brown. Put this in a plate and cover to keep warm.
3. Do this for the second pancake. Serve this with the toffee yogurt. You can

take this with any other low fat yogurt of your choice like vanilla.

Coffee Frappuccino

Ingredients

- For the oat bran galette
- 4 tablespoons of 0% fat Greek yogurt
  4 tablespoons of oat bran
- Your favorite herbs or spices
- 2 whole fresh egg s or fresh egg whites

For the filling

- 2 tablespoons of low fat cream cheese
- Lean cooked meat (ham, beef, chicken or turkey ham)

Instructions

1. Mix all the ingredients in a bowl using a whisk until a smooth batter forms. Add a little yogurt if the batter comes out too thick. Flavor with your favorite spices and/or herbs.

2. Lightly grease the bottom of a non-stick pan and pour half of the batter in. Place the pan over second pancake, place on a plate and cover to keep warm.

3. Slice the galette into two and spread a layer of cream cheese on both sides like with bread. Stuff these with your cooked meat, and serve.

Homemade Yogurt

Ingredients

- 4 teaspoons of sugar-free jelly
- 2 large tub of fat-free natural yogurt
  4 tablespoons of boiling water

Instructions

1. Mix the sugar-free jelly powder with boiling water in a small bowl until it completely dissolves and no lumps are visible at the bottom. Leave this for two minutes to cool down.
2. Blend in the jelly syrup and yogurt in a food processor until they are properly mixed. Use a spoon if you do not have a food processor to mix, but make sure there are no lumps left at the bottom.

3. Instructions using an ice cream machine
4. Pour the jelly mixture and yogurt in the ice cream machine and do as the manual says. This should take less than one hour to get a smooth and gluten free yogurt.
5. Instructions when not using an ice cream machine
6. Pour your mixture into a freezer safe container then cover, and wait for thirty minutes to set.
7. Remove the container from the freezer after thirty minutes, or when it has set and stir thoroughly to break any ice crystals that may have formed and return it to the freezer.
8. Do this every thirty minutes until the frozen yogurt reaches the right consistency.
9. Serve immediately.

10. This is a slightly longer process, and can take up to four hours before the yogurt is ready.

Beef Stew

Ingredients

- 4 roughly chopped celery sticks
- 4 oog of peeled shallots
- 30 /z pint of reduced sodium beef stock 8 sliced chestnut mushrooms
- 2 teaspoon of dried thyme
- 2 bay leaves
- Low fat cooking spray
- 2 teaspoon of dried oregano
- 2 tablespoons of corn flour
- 480g of lean beef strips
- 2 sliced medium carrots
- Freshly ground black pepper

Instructions

1. Pre-heat the oven to i8o degrees C.
2. Place the beef in a bowl, coat with corn flour, and sprinkle freshly ground black pepper.
3. Place shallots, carrots, celery, herbs and mushrooms in a casserole dish and set aside.
4. Take a non-stick pan and spray it with low fat cooking spray at the bottom. Turn the heat to medium high and let the beef cook until it is browned.
5. When done, transfer it to the casserole dish with the vegetable and mix with beef stock.
6. Cover the casserole dish with a lid, place it in the oven, and let it cook for 2 hours or until the meat has cooked well and is tender and the stock becomes thick.

Stuffed Peppers

Ingredients

- 4 tablespoons of oat bran 2 fresh egg
- 2 teaspoon of paprika
- 2 cloves of garlic, crushed
- 4 oog of lean minced beef
- 4 red peppers

Instructions

1. Pre-heat the oven to 450 degrees C.
2. Divide the peppers halfway across their lengths then de-seed and remove any white flesh.
3. Place the peppers in a greaseproof paper lined with a roasting tin and cook until they soften up. This can take about twenty minutes.
4. While these are cooking, prepare your stuffing by putting the fresh egg

, minced beef, 2 tablespoons of oat bran, paprika, and garlic in a food processor and mix. You can mix them in a bowl using a fork if you do not have a food processor.

5. Remove the peppers from the oven, drain excess water and stuff with minced meat mixture.

6. Sprinkle the rest of the oat bran over the peppers and return in the oven to bake for 45 minutes until the meat is done and the oat bran crust turns brown.

Chicken Shirataki Noodle Soup

Ingredients

- 2 teaspoon of fresh grated ginger
- 30 pints of reduced salt chicken stock 2 teaspoon of all spice
- 2 sliced medium courgette
- 450 g of mangetout
- 2oog of pre-packaged or leftover cooked chicken
- 2 tablespoons of low sodium soy sauce
- One 35 og pack of pre-cooked shirataki noodles 2 medium chopped carrot
- Low fat cooking spray
- 4 chopped spring onions
- 4 chopped celery sticks
- 2 tablespoon of corn flour, melted tablespoons of cold water

118

Instructions

1. First, prepare the noodles.
2. Put them in a sink colander, rinse with warm water and then pour in a cooking dish with boiling water for about two minutes.
3. Rinse and put aside.
4. Take a non-stick pan, spray it with low fat cooking spray at the bottom, and cook the celery, carrot, and spring onions under medium heat for about 4 minutes.

5. Mix in the grated ginger while stirring, and let it simmer for some thirty seconds.
6. Add the spice, corn flour, courgette, chicken stock, cooked chicken, mange tout, and simmer for another 50 minutes or until the stock has reduced down and all the vfresh egg ies are tender and cooked.

7. Add the soy sauce and the shirataki noodles then simmer for 2 minutes, and serve!

Arugula Salad

INGREDIENTS

- 2 cups arugula leaves
- 1 cup cranberries
- 1 cup honey
- 1 cup pecans
- 2 cup salad dressing

DIRECTIONS

1. In a bowl combine all ingredients together and mix well
2. Serve with dressing

Masoor Salad

INGREDIENTS

- 1 cup masoor
- 1 cup cucumber
- 2 cup carrot
- 1 cup tomatoes
- 1 cup fresh onion

SALAD DRESSING

- 1 tablespoon olive oil
- 2 tsp lemon juice
- 1 tsp green chillies
- 2 tsp black pepper

DIRECTIONS

1. In a bowl combine all ingredients together and mix well
2. Add salad dressing, toss well and serve

Muskmelon And Pear Salad

INGREDIENTS

- 2 cup pear cubes
- 2 cup apple cubes
- Salad dressing
- 2 cup muskmelon

DIRECTIONS

1. In a bowl combine all ingredients together and mix well
2. Add salad dressing, toss well and serve

Citrus Watermelon Salad

INGREDIENTS

- 2 tsp olive oil
- 2 tsp lemon juice
- 2 tablespoon parsley
- 2 cups watermelon
- 1 cup orange
- 1 cup sweet lime
- 1 cup pomegranate
- SALAD DRESSING

DIRECTIONS

1. In a bowl combine all ingredients together and mix well
2. Add salad dressing, toss well and serve

Potato Salad

INGREDIENTS

- 2 red fresh onion
- 2 cloves garlic
- 1/2 cup lemon juice
- 2 tsp sea salt
- 6 potatoes
- 2 tsp cumin seeds
- 1/2 cup oil
- 2 tsp mustard

DIRECTIONS

1. Steam the potatoes until tender

2. Mix mustard, turmeric powder, lemon juice, cumin seeds, and salt

3. Place the potatoes in a bowl and pour the lemon mixture over

4. Add the chopped fresh onion and minced garlic over

5. Stir to coat and refrigerate covered

6. Add oil and stir before serving

Carrot Salad

INGREDIENTS

- 2 tbs olive oil
- 1/2 lb carrots
- 2 tsp mustard
- 6 tbs lemon juice
- 1/2 tsp salt
- 1 tsp black pepper

DIRECTIONS

1. Mix mustard, lemon juice and oil together
2. Peel and shred the carrots in a bowl
3. Stir in the dressing and season with salt and pepper

4. Mix well and allow to chill for at least 50 minutes

Moroccan Salad

INGREDIENTS

- 4 tbs olive oil
- 2 cloves garlic
- 6 carrots
- 2 tbs lemon juice
- 2 tsp cumin
- 2 tsp paprika
- Salt
- Pepper

DIRECTIONS

1. Peel and slice the carrots
2. Add the carrots in boiled water and simmer for at least 25 minutes

3. Drain and rinse the carrots under cold water

4. Add in a bowl

5. Mix the lemon juice, garlic, cumin, paprika, and olive oil together

6. Pour the mixture over the carrots and toss then season with salt and pepper

7. Serve immediately

Avocado Chicken Salad

INGREDIENTS

- 2 avocado
- 1/2 cup fresh onion
- 2 apple
- 2 cup celery
- 4 tsp lime juice
- 4 tbs cilantro
- 2 chicken breast
- Salt
- Pepper
- Olive oil

DIRECTIONS

1. Dice the chicken breast
2. Season with salt and pepper and cook into a greased skillet until golden
3. Dice the vegetables and place over the chicken in a bowl
4. Mash the avocado and sprinkle in the cilantro
5. Season with salt and pepper and add lime juice
6. Serve drizzled with olive oil

Asparagus Soup

Ingredients:

- Chicken stock
- Nutmeg, a pinch
- Salt and pepper
- Fresh onion, thinly sliced, 2 large
- Asparagus, roughly sliced, 46 0gm
- Olive oil

Instructions:

1. Fry fresh onion in a saucepan coated with olive oil until translucent.
2. Add asparagus and cook for a bit more.
3. Add chicken stock and cook until asparagus is completely cooked.
4. Separate and season with pepper as well as salt.

133

5. Process in nutmeg until smooth before you serve.

Fennel Gratin

Ingredients:

Fennel bulbs, chopped, 2 large

Pepper and salt

Cream cheese, low-fat, 2 tbsp

Cooking oil

Oat bran, 2 tbsp

Instructions:

1. Prepare oven at 450 C.
2. Arrange fennel bulb in a dish and cook for about 50 minutes.
3. Blend in cheese cream and season with salt as well as pepper afterwards.

4. Add cooking oil as well as oat bran; bake for about 50 more minutes or until light brown before you serve.

Cruise Phase Recipes

Chicken and Pepper Casserole
Ingredients:

Vegetable stock, 450 ml

Rosemary, 2 sprig

Salt and pepper to taste

Red pepper, chopped, 2

Corn flour, 2 tsp

Chestnut mushrooms, thickly chopped, 6

Yellow pepper, chopped, 2

Fresh onion, thinly sliced, 2 large

Chicken breast, cubed, 2 large

Olive oil

Instructions:

1. Prepare oven at 450 C.
2. Coat chicken with corn flour.
3. Fry fresh onions in saucepan coated with oil onto medium high heat until translucent.
4. Add chicken and cook until golden.
5. Add pepper as well as mushrooms and simmer for couple more minutes.
6. Add chicken stock and boil.
7. Arrange mixture onto casserole dish; cover with lid and cook for about 425 minutes before you serve.

Chili And Ginger Roast Chicken

Ingredients:

Ginger, peeled, 2 cube

Chicken, 2 medium size.

Lemon, halved, 2

Garlic cloves, 2

Dried oregano, 2 tsp

Paprika, 2 tsp

Red chili pepper, chopped and seeded, 2

Instructions:

1. Prepare oven at 30 0 0 C.
2. Squeeze lemon juice in chicken cavity.
3. Using knife; make hole in chicken for chili, ginger as well as garlic.

138

4. Arrange chicken in roasting tin; add ginger, garlic cloves as well as red chilies.
5. Add sprinkled oregano as well as paprika and cook for about 2 35 minutes or until golden before you serve.

Lemon Chicken

Ingredients:

Garlic clove, chopped, 2 large

Ginger, sliced, 2 cube

Lemon, juiced, 2

Marinade:
Chicken, sliced, 2

Coriander, sliced, handful

Red chili, sliced, 2

Dip:

- Parsley, 2 tbsp
- Salt and pepper
- Chives, sliced, 2 tbsp
- Paprika, 2 tsp
- Greek yogurt, fat-free, 45 0 gm

Instructions:

1. Take a bowl; add all ingredients except chicken and whisk properly to mix.
2. Add sliced chicken in a different bowl; add marinate.
3. Spoon well and let it stand in chiller for about 60 minutes.

Dip:

1. Take a bowl; add all ingredients to it and whisk to mix well.
2. Season with pepper as well as salt and let it chill until chicken is done.
3. Separate chicken from marinate and cook for about 35-40 minutes in oven or until golden before you serve.

Thai Chicken Patties

Ingredients:

Chicken, 480 gm

Coriander, 2 tbsp

Green chili, roughly sliced, 2

Red fresh onion, sliced, 2

Chicken Patties:
Garlic clove, sliced, 2

Ginger, peeled and sliced, 2 small

Dip:

Spring onions, sliced, 4

Lemon juice

Greek yogurt, 45 0 gm

Chives, sliced, 2 tbsp

Salt and pepper

Instructions:

1. In food processor; add all ingredients and process well until smooth.
2. Arrange in a bowl and season with salt as well as pepper.
3. Cover and let it stand in refrigerator to chill.

Thai patties:

1. Except chicken; add all ingredients to a food processor and process until smooth.
2. Combine mixture as well as chicken thoroughly and make patties.
3. Add patties to non-stick pan coated with oil and cook for about 35

minutes on medium-high heat or
until light brown.
4. Serve alongside dip.

Steak Pizzaiola

Ingredients:

Tomato paste, 2 tbsp

Garlic cloves, chopped, 2

Lean beef

Parsley, sliced, handful

Cooking spray

Instructions:

1. Add beef to saucepan coated with cooking spray.
2. Daub paste around chicken after diluting by adding water.
3. Add half sliced parsley as well as garlic and cook for about 50 minutes on medium-high heat.
4. Add a bit hot water if sauce is thick.
5. Season with black pepper and serve with remaining sprinkled sliced parsley.

Mini Burgers

Ingredients:

Garlic cloves, sliced, 2 small

Oat bran, 2 tbsp

Cajun spice mix, 2 tbsp

Green chili, sliced, 2 (optional)

Chicken breast, minced, 6 00 gm

Fresh egg , 2

Instructions:

1. In a food processor; add all ingredients together and process well to form batter.
2. Make burgers from the batter.
3. Place burgers onto pre-heated griddle pan and cook onto high heat until done.
4. Enjoy alongside yogurt.

Rosemary Beef Burgers

Ingredients:

Burger:
Nutmeg, 2 tsp

Oat bran, 4 tbsp

Black pepper

Rosemary, sliced, 2 tbsp

Lean beef, minced, 470 gm

Fresh egg , 2

Dip:

Dried dill, 2 tsp

Yogurt, 45 0 gm

Smoked paprika, 2 tsp

Instructions:

1. Take a bowl; add all dip ingredients and blend.
2. Cover and let it chill in refrigerator.

Burger:

1. In a food processor; add all burger ingredients and blend until smooth to form batter.
2. Arrange batter onto griddle pan and cook onto high heat until golden before you serve.

Salmon Baked Omelet

Ingredients:

Fresh egg s, 6

Smoked, salmon, sliced, 300 gm

Dried dill, 2 tbsp

Chives, sliced, 2 tbsp

Yogurt, fat-free, 2 tbsp

Black pepper

Instructions:

1. Prepare oven at 450 C.
2. Take a bowl; add 2/4 of sliced salmon, yogurt, fresh fresh egg as well as dried dill, combine and season with pepper.
3. Decant mixture in a tin and add remaining salmon topping.

150

4. Add sliced chives as well and bake for about 50-55 minutes before you serve.

Cottage Pie

Ingredients

- 4 carrots: 2 chopped finely for the pie filling, and 4 chopped roughly for the mash topping
- 2 finely chopped onion
- 4^{00}g lean beef mince or turkey mince 4 finely chopped celery sticks
- 2 teaspoon of dried thyme 2 tablespoons of tomato paste 2 teaspoon of marjoram

- ^{2} teaspoon of dried rosemary
- 2 teaspoons of corn flour, melted in 2 tablespoons of cold water
- 2 pint of reduced salt beef stock Low fat cooking spray
- 2 swede, cut into chunks
- Salt and pepper

Instructions

1. Put the swede and roughly chopped carrots in a deep pan then add boiling water and leave to simmer. Meanwhile, prepare the cottage pie filling.
2. Spray the bottom of a non-stick pan with low fat cooking pan then put the chopped onion and let it cook under medium heat until it turns golden brown.

3. Add the celery, finely chopped carrot, and 4 tablespoons of hot water. Leave it for another three minutes.

4. Add the tomato paste, beef mince, and herbs, and salt and pepper to taste. You may add 2 tablespoon of Italian herb mix if you like. Cook for ten minutes or until the meat is almost set.

5. Add beef stock topping and corn flour mixed with water.

6. Simmer for another 45 minutes or until the stock has reduced down.

7. Drain the carrot and Swede, and mush them well. Spoon-feed the cottage pie filling into two microwaveable dishes then add the carrot mash mixture and season with freshly ground black pepper.

8. Let these cook under the grill for about twenty minutes if you are eating right away, or put them in the

fridge for later use, but be sure to cover with a cling film.

CPSIA information can be obtained
at www.ICGtesting.com
Printed in the USA
BVHW071714110321
602278BV00011B/847

9 781990 207754